Foster's Opioid Classification Addiction Status (FOCAS) Guide

Determining Opioid Users Status and Treatment Options

D. TERRENCE FOSTER, M.D.

Foster's Opioid Classification Addiction Status (FOCAS) Guide

Determining Opioid Users Status and Treatment Options

D. TERRENCE FOSTER, M.D., FAAPMR, DABPM

Global Health and Consortium Publishing.

GHC^P

Foster's Opioid Classification Addiction Status (FOCAS) Guide

Copyright © 2018 by D Terrence Foster

Publisher: Global Health and Consortium
PO Box 824, Morrow, GA 30260.

GHCPublishing.com
GHC^P

Printed in the United States of America. No claim to Original United States Government Work.

First published in January 2019.

Library of Congress Cataloging in Publication Data

Foster's Opioid Classification Addiction Status Guide:

D Terrence Foster, M.D.

1SBN 13: 978-1-7328804-3-6 (Paperback).

Library of Congress Control Number: 2018912204

Also available:

1SBN 13: 978-1-7328804-4-3 (eBook).

Disclaimer

This publication is intended to inform and educate consumers and medical providers in general. The subject matter that is discussed encompasses many areas related to the Opioids use as well as specific disciplines that are associated or incorporated in the subject matter. Also, the subject matter continues to change and evolves, because of these reasons and others the readers are advised to consult with their own personnel for medical and or legal advice when appropriate.

The author has taken great care in researching and presenting the facts that are in this book. Every effort has been made to ensure that this book is free of error. Regardless of that, however, the author and publisher do not assume any responsibilities or liabilities for errors or omission. Also, all liabilities are disclaimed from using any or part of the information from this book.

For the references and recommended reading that are listed, every effort has been made to obtain and give credits for all the material that we use that required copyright release and even those that did not. If for any reason any content that appears in this book does not have the author's or publishers' permission, we apologized for the error of omission and asked that you, please contact us for corrective action.

Dedication

To all my patients over the years who I am privileged to treat, and whom I have allowed to teach me.

Foster's Opioid Classification Addiction Status (FOCAS) Guide

Acknowledgments

The writing of this book is a collaboration of many different forces coming together. I want to take the opportunity to thank my beloved wife Maxine, who shared in the sacrifice of this project coming to completion and also my present staff (CPARM and Personal Injury Solutions) particularly our practice administrator Mrs. Arlene Soriano. I have learned a lot from you all and continued to learn. You have helped to provide clarity even when I am at my best.

If I sometimes seem unmoved, unshakable and display a sense of calmness even in what may be considered as chaotic, it is because of the many great teachers I have had both as a student and as a professional. Over the years I have also learned from my former students, colleagues, but most of all from countless patients that I have allowed to teach me. The medical profession is a never-ending and growing Web of knowledge; I am so grateful for the power of learning and so many who have contributed to my growth.

Some of the references are from the governmental press or publication releases, research or data collections. I find it necessary to give special thanks to the many great scientists and researchers and assistants who work in government agencies. Without their work, many of the things that we do today would not be possible. I am truly grateful.

There are no commercial or sponsoring entity or relevant conflicting disclosure associated with this book.

Table of Contents

INTRODUCTION

What is this book about?

The opioid epidemic according to the Centers for Disease and Control Prevention was responsible for 632,000 deaths between the years 1999 and 2016. Sixty-six percent of these deaths involved opioids; the rest were none opioids drugs. 40% of the opioid deaths were attributed to legally prescribed opioids, and the other 60% was from illegal drugs such as heroin and illicitly manufactured fentanyl. For the year 2017, it is projected that over 72,000 people will die from drug overdose. Of this number, about 49,000 will die from opioids. Statistics like these make the opioid epidemic one of the most significant epidemics in our modern era.

As clinicians and healthcare providers we are always faced with the need to treat, provide supportive care, psychosocial services among other related services to individuals who are confronted with the challenges of the opioid epidemic or just the need to start opioid treatment. We will see users of opioids at different levels of treatments, different needs, and at various levels of risk and potential for overdose. This is in part the need for this book and its primary objective. The title of the book is:

The Foster's Opioid Classification Addiction Status (FOCAS) Guide

It detailed a nomenclature (naming) or grouping of every one of us into a class. This will allow for easier characterization of individuals/patients or potential users and users of opioids. There is a flowchart (algorithm) /table that is constructed that will enable comparable language and descriptions among providers in the healthcare field. Once this is understood this algorithm/ table can also help with treatment stratification or protocols. In general, this has the potential to simplify communications between professionals.

This classification is not a risk assessment tool for the use of opioids. However, understanding patients' addiction status will allow for better stratification concerning treatment options and possibly the level of care and intervention each patient or individual may need. Throughout the algorithm, patients' risk level will vary and change and may be at any level regardless of the group or class they entered or are classified.

Appropriate medical, nonmedical intervention, treatment and the possible obstacles that will be faced by those of us who work with chronic and acute pain patients can be more clearly defined once we have an understanding and knowledge of each one's Opioid Addiction Status.

What this book provides is a relatively simple but a useful approach to a very complex problem, as well as providing information that will create a better understanding among healthcare providers/physicians that will allow uniform communications among professionals involved with the opioids use, treatment and addiction.

Who Should Read This Book and Why?

This book will be very useful to anyone involved in a health care capacity or service related areas. These include but not limited to medical doctors/providers, physician assistant, nurse practitioners, nurses, counselors, therapists, aids to these professionals, community leaders, coaches, providers of Addiction Medicine support and treatment services and finally parents and family members who are interested in the opioid classification status of anyone even if they're not being treated.

I strongly recommend that those who use the information contained, please expand on your knowledge by continue reading, some of the references that are provided in this book, which will start the process for you. Also, I have written a comprehensive book on the opioid epidemic titled: **The Opioid Epidemic Consumers & Healthcare Guide** which is likely to be very helpful.

What Makes Me Think I Can Write a Book Like This?

Finally, I decided to write this book because of the knowledge that I've acquired in the field of health care and particular medicine after practicing as a medical doctor for more than 20 years.

I decided to write this book when I was writing the book titled: **The Opioid Epidemic Consumers and Healthcare Guide.** I realized that I could not find any classification of opioids use that would allow me to present the opioid epidemic in a cohesive and meaningful way. FOCAS was created to streamlined the framework of that book.

Concerning my credential, I am Board Certified in Physical Medicine and Rehabilitation as well as Board Certified in Pain Medicine. I am still practicing and am the Chief Medical Officer of a Licensed Pain Clinic where Addiction Medicine and treating patients with addiction is also part of our practice. I previously served as the Medical Director for an Acute Inpatient Rehabilitation Center for ten years. That center had a considerable number of the patients that I treated that had significant acute pain as well as chronic pain.

In addition, I have also worked in Skilled Nursing Facilities for several years caring for the elderly. Besides, I must say that I have been truly fortunate to have passed through some of the most excellent institutions of learning that any physician could have asked for in a lifetime.

It is my intention that this book will make a difference in helping healthcare providers and service workers in the field of pain management and addiction medicine as well as others in service-related areas and making the process of treatment easier with commonalities of fundamental knowledge.

CHAPTER ONE

FOSTER'S OPIOID CLASSIFICATION ADDICTION STATUS (FOCAS) GUIDE

The Foster's Opioid Classification Addiction Status (**FOCAS**) is a nomenclature (naming) or grouping of every one of us into a class. This allows for easier characterization of individuals/patients or potential users and users of opioids. This flowchart (algorithms) will enable comparable language and descriptions among providers in the healthcare field. This can also help with treatment stratification or protocols. In general, this has the potential to simplify communications between professionals as well as between professionals and their patients.

The treatment protocols for pain adapted for patients will vary depending on the chronicity or acuteness of those conditions being treated as well as the complexity of them and any other medical conditions (comorbidities) that may affect the outcome of the treatment. Multiple non-opioids regiments are often used in the treatment of pain conditions often before opioids are introduced. These may include but are not limited to anti-inflammatory medications, non-opioid analgesics, anti-spasmodic medications, and mood stabilizers. Patients may be required to be involved in physical therapy, psychiatric care, behavioral therapy; or incorporate therapeutic modalities to enhance the treatment protocol.

There are numerous bodies/organizations such as the CDC, the VA, Multiple Medical Associations and countless other institutions have proposed and or published guidelines for treatment for patients that have acute as well as chronic pain.[4,5,6]

In an effort to understand the context in which individuals who present with pain are treated at different levels I have created a flowchart (algorithm) to assist the healthcare providers and even readers to better understand the various path to recovery and or addiction. This is called the **Foster's Opioid Classification Addiction Status (FOCAS) .**

THE FLOWCHART (ALGORITHM) FOR FOCAS GUIDE
FOSTER'S OPIOID ADDICTION CLASSIFICATION STATUS (FOACS)

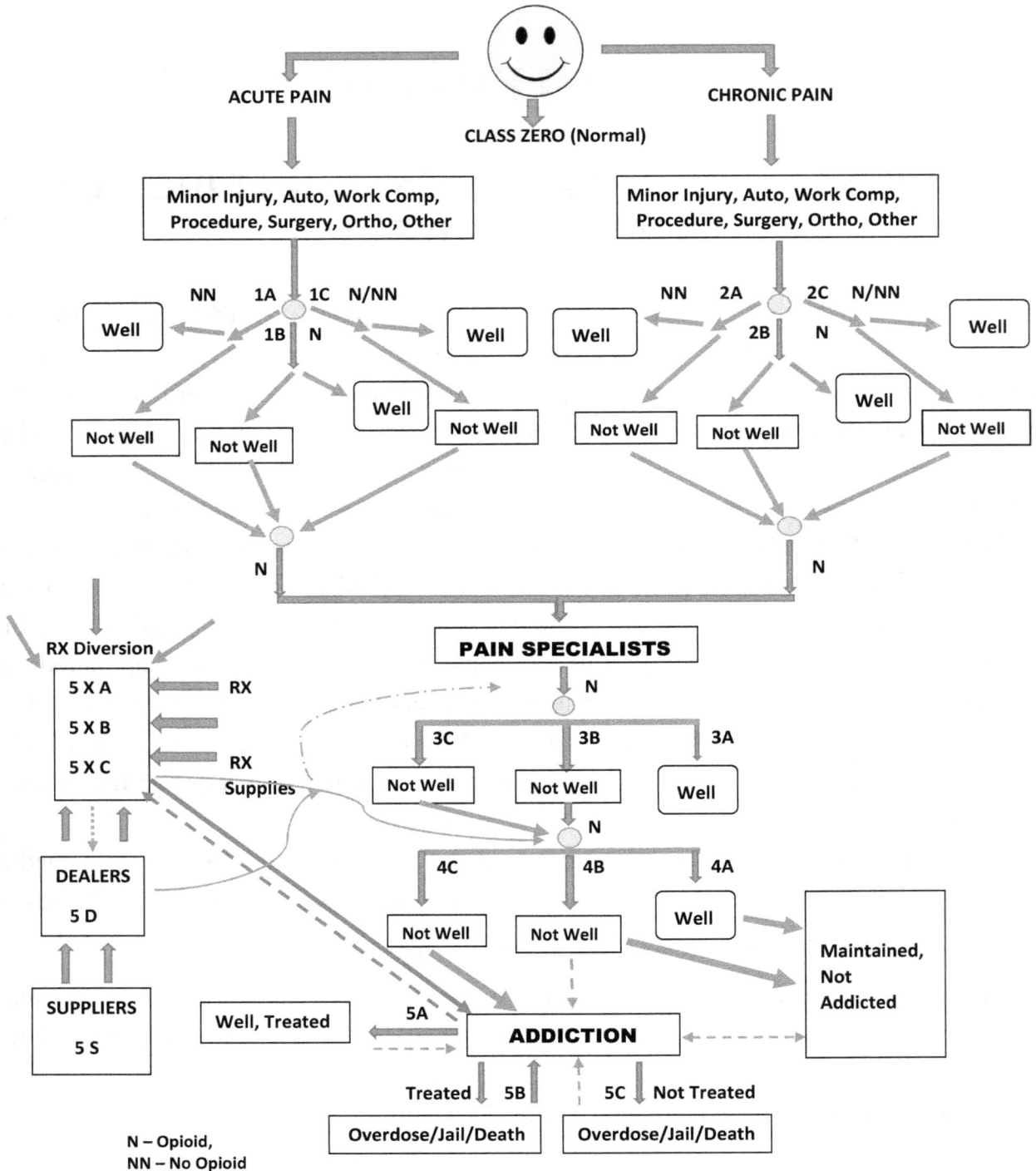

ACUTE PAIN

CLASS ZERO (Normal)

CHRONIC PAIN

Minor Injury, Auto, Work Comp, Procedure, Surgery, Ortho, Other

Minor Injury, Auto, Work Comp, Procedure, Surgery, Ortho, Other

NN 1A 1C N/NN

Well   1B N   Well

Well   Not Well

Not Well   Not Well   Well   Not Well

NN 2A 2C N/NN

Well   2B N   Well

Not Well   Not Well   Well   Not Well

N

N

PAIN SPECIALISTS

N

RX Diversion

5 X A
5 X B
5 X C

RX

RX
Supplies

3C   3B   3A

Not Well   Not Well   Well

N

4C   4B   4A

Not Well   Not Well   Well

DEALERS

5 D

SUPPLIERS

5 S

Well, Treated

5A

Maintained, Not Addicted

ADDICTION

Treated   5B   5C   Not Treated

Overdose/Jail/Death   Overdose/Jail/Death

N – Opioid,
NN – No Opioid

20

REGARDING FOSTER'S OPIOID CLASSIFICATION ADDICTION STATUS (FOCAS)

1. **Class 0, 1 and 2** are opioid naïve, these are users with no opioid use or limited opioid use such as prior prescriptions for minor procedures that resulted in small quantities of opioids prescribed (example: from dentists, podiatrists, etc.)

2. **Class 3** has a history of opioid use, with initial intervention by consultants, they are not addicted to opioids, some may have developed tolerance.

3. **Class 4** has extended opioids use with or without specialists, some of them may have opioid tolerance or dependence.

4. **Class 5** this class has the **Addiction Groups 5A, 5B and 5C** (Addicts or Opioid Use Disorder groups), the **Illegal Groups 5XA, 5XB and 5XC**, as well as the **Dealers Groups 5XD (A, B, and C)**, and **Suppliers Groups 5XS (A, B, and C)**.

5. The group designated as "C" has a history of psychiatric, psychological, behavioral disorder, cognitive impairment or non-opioids substance abuse history in Groups One and Two. However, Classes 3 and 4 are combinations of the preceding Classes. Therefore, Groups 3A and 4A, (well groups) now have patients previously designated as "C" in Groups One and Two (patients with psychiatric disorders/substance abuse, etc. do get well and can be stable on or off opioids). Groups 3B, 4B, 5A and 5B are the treated groups without psychiatric, cognitive or non-opioid substance abuse disorders.

6. Treatments referred to range from limited therapy and or medications to multidisciplinary approach intervention and or medications.

7. There are multiple overlaps and when in doubt patients should be placed at the higher level (more complex) with respect to treatment and classification.

8. Most of the addictions, overdoses and opioid deaths that occur in the United States are likely to come from the Groups 5XA, 5XB, and 5XC. These are primarily the none prescription opioids (diverted legally prescribed opioids) and illegal opioids such as heroin and illicitly manufactured fentanyl. It may sometimes be difficult to establish wellness accurately with respect to 5XA and 5XB and 5XC in general.

9.   If the drugs dealers and suppliers become users of illegal opioids and or illegal non-opioid drugs their classification will be 5XD (A, B or C) and 5XS (A, B or C) respectively.

The associated table referred to as the **FOCAS TABLE** on the next page also explains the flowchart.

FOCAS TABLE

Time	Class	Groups		
None	**ZERO**	-	Normal	-
Less than three mo., acute opioid naïve	**ONE**	**1A:** treatment without opioids, well	**1B:** treatment with opioids	**1C:** treatment with or without opioids, psychiatry, etc.
3 mo. -1yr plus, chronic opioid naïve	**TWO**	**2A:** treatment without opioids, well	**2B:** treatment with opioids	**2C:** treatment with or without an opioid, psych., etc.
1-2 yrs., chronic, opioids	**THREE**	**3A:** treatment with opioids, well	**3B:** treatment with opioids, not well	**3C:** treatment, well, not well, psych, etc.
>2yrs, chronic, opioids	**FOUR**	**4A:** treatment with opioids, well	**4B:** treatment with opioids, not well	**4C:** treatment, not well, psych, etc.
>2yrs, chronic, opioids	**FIVE (Addiction groups, use illicit opioids/Rx)**	**5A**: well, not well. Usually have good support, money/social network	**5B:** well, not well, OD, jail. Have some level of support.	**5C:** not well, Psych, etc. No treatment, OD, jail, death? Have poor support structure.
Undefined	**FIVE (Illicit Groups)**	**These are the groups with multiple unknown factors** Without medical doctors/services or sense of direction Extremely difficult to treat, numerous unknown factors. Very risky.		
	X	**5XA**	Has no pain, using illegal prescription drugs	
	X	**5XB**	Has pain, using illegal prescription drugs	
	X	**5XC**	Has pain or no pain, using illegal prescription & illegal none-prescription drug, psychiatry, etc.	
	X	**5XD (A, B or C)**	Illegal Drug dealers	
	X	**5XS (A, B or C)**	Illegal Drug suppliers	

UNDERSTANDING THE CLASSIFICATION

Acute Treatments Opioids and None-opioid

Patients present to their healthcare providers very often with either acute pain or chronic pain. **Acute pain,** defined as pain which will typically resolve in about three months; and **chronic pain,** which lasts longer than three months.

Acute pain may be the result of minor injuries, automobile accidents, workers compensation-related accident/injuries, or procedures such as surgeries by various specialists: orthopedic, dental, podiatry, etc. Others may have nonspecific pain, for example, in the stomach, ear, or headaches.

Patients with acute pain injuries and/or surgical procedures would fall into **Class 1: Groups 1 A, 1B and 1C** if they have never taken or have only used opioids minimally in the past (example: small quantities of opioids with a few days' duration, given by dentists and other specialists), or are so-called naïve patients. Depending on the severity of their injuries or procedures, they may be started on non-narcotics as a first-line treatment, as recommended by the CDC guidelines and others.[4] However, some of these patients are started on opioids; again, this depends on the severity and type of injuries/procedures.

Other factors that dictate what these patients are started on are the medical providers and the treatment options they have available or are capable of administering. One could reasonably justify the need for opioids in someone who had an amputated limb as opposed to someone who sprained one of the joints in their extremity. The big questions are often: how long is it appropriate to continue opioids particularly for someone who has a significant injury, or underwent a major surgery? Is a seven-day prescription enough, and if not, how much longer? And during that course, how much medication is considered appropriate? Very often, the patients who did not respond to non-opioid therapeutic intervention would have continued on opioids and entered into the chronic phase of pain management.

The providers at this point will have to decide on whether or not they want to keep treating the patient and managing their opioids/pain management needs.

Patients in **Class 2: Groups 2A, 2B, and 2C** sometimes with minor injuries become chronic pain patients and, in some instances, would have been given more opioids than is appropriate. These patients would join the chronic opioid-naïve patients who have failed to respond to non-opioids or opioids in the initial phase of treatment.

It is worth mentioning that, there are other factors that sometimes cause some patients to go from being an acute status to chronic. Some of these patients may be involved in automobile accidents/personal injury, workers compensation injury and other litigation pending injuries. Because of potential secondary gain and pending unsettled cases, some of these patients may continue to take opioids even though their condition may not justify the need. Other patients also who may have secondary gains are patients who are on disability and need to "remain sick" in order to keep validating the need for disability.

Chronic Treatment with Opioids

The vast majority of patients that have now become chronic pain patients in their early stage they were treated by primary care, family practitioner internal medicine and to some lesser extent surgical specialties.

Now in general over 50% of the opioids that are prescribed in the United States are prescribed by primary care physicians, family practice and internal medicine physicians or providers. Sometime it might be years before some of these patients are referred to **Pain Management Specialists**; At that stage, they are either in **Class 3 or 4** and in some instance heading into **Class 5**. This class has the **Addiction Groups 5A, 5B and 5C**, the **Illegal Groups 5XA, 5XB and 5XC**, as well as the **Dealers Groups 5XD (A, B, and C), and Suppliers Groups 5XS (A, B, and C).**

Most of the discussions about opioid overdose deaths, in general, is centered around those that do not have an opioid dependence or an opioid use disorder – addiction. This is a reasonable thing to do even though opioid addiction is also very important.

The reality is that almost all patients are users of opioids that died from overdose were at some point in their initial, and early stage of use were considered "safe" before they become opioid dependence or addicts - opioids use disorder patients. Prevention and early intervention processes are significantly easier to manage than opioid addiction thereby reducing the risks of progression. However, those that have an opioid dependence and or addiction to opioids are at higher risks of dying than those without even though overall there are fewer of them than are none-addicted individuals. Non-addicted patients or individuals have died and continued to die from opioids overdose, so it is important to know that users of opioids do not have to be opioid dependence or opioid addicts for them to die of an overdose.

According to the NIH publication in 2015 about two million people suffer from substance use disorder related to opioid prescriptions. Of the total number of users of opioids, it is estimated that 8 to 12% will develop an opioid use disorder.[6]

The challenges that are faced by some of these treating physicians/providers is that they either have limited options to offer pain patients other than medications or they have additional options but failed to use them.

The patients on the other hand when they present to pain specialists on high-dose opioids are expecting to have a similar treatment as they did with their primary care providers. Often once this desire is not fulfilled, they are either discharge because of being noncompliant, or they leave on their own accord to go shopping somewhere that they believe will meet their opioids needs. Eventually, they are likely to get to a point where no one is able or willing to prescribe the amount of opioids they need, so they then end up seeking supplementation from illegal drugs like heroin and illicit synthetic opioids analogs. This often continues on a downward spiral course if intervention and treatment are not initiated in a timely and aggressive manner.

Treatment of Users of Illegal Opioids

Sixty percent of all opioids related overdose deaths are directly related to users of illegal opioids such as heroin and illicitly manufactured fentanyl. 40% of opioids related deaths are due to legally prescribed opioids.

Users of illegal opioids fall into three broad groups in **Class 5X,** classified as **Group 5XA, 5XB, and 5XC.** Members of these groups are usually functioning or operating without any or very limited healthcare, social service or direct medical care or supervision. Sometimes if any service is available, it probably is unrelated to their opioid substance abuse or needs.

Group 5XA: these are individuals who have no medical problem in general and are simply using the drugs for personal use or just experimenting. This group has the lowest average age, often comprised of teenagers and young adults. They may have obtained the opioids from someone's medicine cabinets, given to them by a friend usually free in the first few instances. They may also have received their first trial of opioids from cheap, available illegal heroin or illicitly manufactured fentanyl. This may have simply started as "just try this" it will make you feel better. This can and will often lead to the unaware unsuspecting users become addicted on the opioids or even in the early introduction stage leads to deaths by overdose.

This group of users often surprised their family and loved ones because they are generally considered "the best of society" which has everything to gain and nothing to lose. However, once this naïve user of illicit opioids become addicted and the free supplies of legally prescribed opioids or illegally free opioids are no longer available for free than these victims become slaves to their opioid craving, "dependence/addictions" and their suppliers.

Group 5XB: these are individuals who do have a medical problem involving chronic pain without psychiatric disorder or other illegal substance abuse. They have failed to continue to get medical care, because of expenses such as no health care insurance or have noncompliant issues with previous legally prescribed pain management providers. They now resort to obtaining medications from diversion prescriptions, and subsequently, once that is unavailable, they will resort to less expensive illegal drugs such as heroin, or illicitly manufactured fentanyl or designer/analog drugs presume to be opioids. These patients generally may fall in the range from opioid tolerance to full-blown opioid use disorder – addicts.

Group 5XC: the users in this group are comprised of patients who have a history of or have developed mental disorders, related cognitive issues and/or substance abuse issues. Their drug of choice is not necessarily opioids, but are related to illegal drugs such as cocaine, methamphetamine, PCP, etc., or they may have substance abuse problems related to alcohol or benzos, etc. These users may or may not have had pain when they started using illegal opioids or legal opioids obtained illegally.

They will obtain their opioid similar to those in **Groups 5XA and 5XB**; from diversion or illegal opioids supplies. Their path is similar. However, their course to recovery and treatment are often much more difficult because it is compounded by their underlying psychiatric, mental or substance abuse related issues. Unfortunately, mental illness is one of many categories in healthcare that is generally underserved. Many patients will go undiagnosed for an extended period, or even those that are diagnosed with mental disorder or illness may get only limited or no treatment for their conditions.

It is easy to see that someone has a problem if he or she is carried into your office with blood all over the place and broken bone sticking out of one of his or her extremities. However, it may not be easy to believe or recognize that someone who walks into your office smiling accompanied by a caring spouse or caregiver may have an even more significant problem.

Groups 5XD and 5XS: are designated groups of individuals that are involved in opioids as dealers and suppliers. Their faith is often difficult to determine and will fall into any of the **Class 5** categories once they become users, classified as **Groups 5XD (A, B, or C)** and **Groups 5XS (A, B, or C).** In order to effectively treats these groups of users that I have described as "**Users of Illegal Opioids,**" they will almost always need a multidisciplinary approach to their treatment. One of the greatest challenges in these categories is that there are so many unknown factors, most of which are unlikely to be known prior to or during treatment. However, it goes without saying that this group will remain the most significant challenge for all of us who care about opioid addiction and finding meaningful solutions. This group overall now accounts for more than 40% of all drugs overdose deaths in the country. It is also the fastest rising group of any drug-related overdose deaths.

Drug-related deaths from other non-opioids cause account for about 34% and drugs related deaths related to legal prescriptions overdose accounts for about 26%. Early indicators are this number (40%) will continue to increase as the spread of cheap heroin, illicitly manufactured fentanyl and other designer/ analog drugs continue to be a significant percentage of the illegal opioids available for all to use.[7.8]

Comparing FOCAS with Other Scales or Classifications

There have been many different scales and classifications that providers have been using in medicine to help categorize or simplify protocols, improve nomenclatures, help to streamline treatments among other things. Some of these are based on research; others are non-research based. However, they are constructed in various forms in many different areas or disciplines of medicine and science in general. I will briefly examine and discuss a few of them that are likely to be familiar to healthcare workers or providers. One thing that is almost universally true is that, although they may be helpful, they are not perfect, and in some cases have very limited use. This is in part due to the fact that the data or information that is gathered from the subjects is often subject dependent, which means that we are relying on the person being examined to be truthful and honest and not try to deceive the examiner. Hence, the conclusion one can draw or compute from these scales or classifications may not be a true representation of the subject been examined. This at best often creates what can be described as a semi-objective assessment which again although useful must be taken in contexts of the total examination of the patients or subjects.

Manual Muscle Testing

The Manual Muscle Testing Scale ranges from 0 to 5. This test relies on the patient' participation; if we're trying to determine how strong or weak a particular muscle or group of muscles are, for example, the patient's hand grip, the patient has the option of how strong he or she wants the grip strength to be if there is no abnormality.

If on the other hand, the patient has specific neurological deficits which make his or her hand grip objectively weaker let's say 4/5, then he or she can by his or her action determine how strong the hand grip is up to 4/5. However, he or she cannot test more than 4/5 even if the intent is there.

Opioid Risk Tool

Opioid Risk Tool (ORT) is one of the most widely used risk assessment tools in pain management. Patients who know how the scores are calculated can and will give the answers that they know will modify the results the provider can obtain. For example, patients who have family members who have a past history of illicit drugs, prescription drugs and/or alcohol abuse may deny all of these, as well as denying the same for themselves. Therefore, these patients may be considered to be very low risk just by being able to deny theirs and their families' history while in fact, they would be very high-risk patients if they correctly answered the questions as required.[3]

Ashworth and Modified Ashworth Scales

Ashworth and Modified Ashworth Scales have some similarities to Manual Muscle Testing. However, it has a greater probability of obtaining more reliable and objective results, particularly when someone with moderate to significant neurological impairment (Spasticity) is being tested. The scales range from 0 to 4 and 0 to 5 respectively (or both 0-4 depending on plus added), it is also more examiner dependent compared to Manual Muscle Testing.

Glasgow Coma Scale

The Glasgow Coma Scale is used to assess patients in a coma (original use), now use to assess all acute medical and trauma patients' level of consciousness. Scores range 3-15, patients with scores of 3-8 are usually considered to be in a coma. There is still room for patients' modification or results that is patient dependent or control such as **localized painful stimuli**; that is a purposeful movement where the stimulus is applied, or patients' **ability to obey commands** such as being able to do simple things that are asked of them. This, of course, would be applicable to patients that are not comatose.

There are indeed numerous other classifications, scales or tests, like these above. There use must be administered in the contexts of the patients' objective findings, as well as the clinical judgment of the providers considering all factors in determining the best way to proceed in managing their patients. FOCAS will fall in the same general category.

FOCAS Timeline. The timeline indicated for acute pain, chronic pain and the effect of long-term use of opioids have been documented in the literature, although there is not an extensive amount of research that has been done in this area. One research article in part looked at the long-term effect and benefits of opioids used to treat acute and chronic opioids use for at least one year, the second article followed noncancer patients for up to 13 years who were treated with opioids, some of whom died from opioid-related overdose who had a median 2.6 years from when they first receive opioid prescription.[1,2]

References

1. Chou R, Deyo R, Devine B, et al. The effectiveness and risks of long-term opioid treatment of chronic pain. Evidence Report/Technology Assessment No. 218. AHRQ Publication No. 14-E005-EF. Rockville, MD: Agency for Healthcare Research and Quality; 2014 https://effectivehealthcare.ahrq.gov/sites/default/files/pdf/chronic-pain-opioid-treatment_research.pdf. Last accessed November 10, 2018.

2. Eric Kaplovitch, Tara Gomes, Ximena Camacho, Irfan A. Dhalla, Muhammad M. Mamdani, David N. Juurlink. Sex Differences in Dose Escalation and Overdose Death during Chronic Opioid Therapy: A Population-Based Cohort Study. August 20, 2015. https://journals.plos.org/plosone/article?id=10.1371/journal.pone.0134550Last accessed November 10, 2018.

3. Lynn R. Webster, MD, and Rebecca M. Webster. Predicting Aberrant Behaviors in Opioid-Treated Patients: Preliminary Validation of the Opioid Risk Tool. Pain Medicine 6 (6), 432-442, 2005 http://pcssnow.org/wp-content/uploads/2014/11/ORT.pdf Accessed October 6, 2018

4. Deborah Dowell, MD; Tamara M. Haegerich, Ph.D.; Roger Chou, MD. CDC Guideline for Prescribing Opioids for Chronic Pain —the United States, 2016. March 18, 2016. https://www.cdc.gov/mmwr/ volumes/65/rr/rr6501e1.htm. Accessed March 7, 2018.

5. VA/DoD Clinical Practice Guideline for Opioid Therapy for Chronic Pain. Department of Veterans Affairs Department of Defense. February 2017. https://www.healthquality.va.gov/guidelines/Pain/cot/ VADoDOTCPG022717.pdf. Accessed March 7, 2018.

6. National Institute on Drug Abuse. Principles of Drug Addiction Treatment: A Research-Based Guide. Third edition. Last reviewed December 2012. https://www.drugabuse.gov/sites/default/files/ podat_1.pdf. Accessed July 2, 2018.

7. The Centers for Disease Control and Prevention. Understanding the Epidemic. https://www.cdc.gov/drugoverdose/epidemic/index.html. Last visited June 16, 2018.

8. Puja Seth, Ph.D.; Lawrence Scholl, Ph.D.; Rose A. Rudd, MSPH; Sarah Bacon, Ph.D., *MMMWR*. Overdose deaths involving opioids, cocaine, and psychostimulants – the United States, 2015 – 2016. https://www.cdc.gov/mmwr/volumes/67/wr/mm6712a1.htm. Accessed May 5, 2018.

CHAPTER TWO

Case Studies – Examples and Use of FOCAS

This section contains examples of cases of patients which are used to provide clarity for the application of FOCAS. Each case is followed by sets of relevant questions that are in a workbook format. The classification/answer to the case is provided after the questions.

CASE # ONE

Mr. RY is a 54-year-old male who was involved in a motor vehicle accident approximately one week ago. He presented at an office complaining of neck pain back pain as well as pain affecting his mouth. He was a passenger in a vehicle driven by his son when the vehicle he was in was hit from behind by another vehicle. His pain ranges from 7 to 10 and is essentially constant.

He previously had no complaint of pain involving his back, neck or mouth. He is currently taking no medications. He denies illicit drugs use. He also denies ever been involved in any previous accident or any incident relating to the cause of any pain. He has no apparent cognitive deficits.

Treatment: He was started on a non-opioid regimen along with therapy, chiropractic care/physical therapy.

QUESTIONS:

Type of Pain Acute/ Chronic: _____ *Duration of Pain* _____

Psychosocial Comorbidities _____

Cognitive Impairment _____

Opioids Medications _____

Length of Time on Opioids Medications _____

*Prior Treatments Received for the
Condition* _____

Providers Pain management _____
Psychiatrist/Behavioral/Addiction

_____

Psychosocial /financial Support _____

Others _____

ANSWER - CASE # ONE

Class _____1_____ Group _____A_____

FOCAS: 1A

Comments: Mr. RY pain is acute in nature, with no prior chronic pain or use of opioids, he would fall into **Class I and Group A.**

CASE # TWO

Patient DP is a 30-year-old female who was involved in a motor vehicle accident approximately ten days ago resulting in low back pain and left shoulder pain. She was seen in the emergency room and was started on Tylenol # 3 and anti-inflammatory as well as a muscle relaxer. She presented at an office with pain which she stated is constant and is at a 10 out of 10. She is employed as a car detailer and has missed work since accidents. She denies being involved in any other accident or incident resulting in trauma or pain. She denies any use of illegal drugs, any psychiatric illness or treatment in the past. No cognitive deficit appreciated.

Treatment: the patient was started on a muscle relaxer, extra strength Tylenol 3 to 4 times a day and ibuprofen. She was also referred for therapy – physical/chiropractic

QUESTIONS:

Type of Pain Acute/ Chronic: _____ *Duration of Pain* _____

Psychosocial Comorbidities _____

Cognitive Impairment _____

Opioids Medications _____

Length of Time on Opioids Medications _____

Prior Treatments Received for the Condition _____

Providers Pain management _____
Psychiatrist/Behavioral/Addiction _____

Psychosocial /financial Support _____

Others _____

ANSWER - CASE # TWO

Class _____1_____ Group _____B_____

FOCAS: 1B

Comments: This case is very similar to case number one, although the patient was restarted on extra strength Tylenol, she still remains **Class 1 and Group B** having had no opioids before. If the patient was not prescribed opioids she would have been classified as belonging to **Group 1A.**

CASE # THREE

Patient KR is an 87-year-old female who has low back pain, right shoulder pain and bilateral knee pain for several years. She stated that she tried to avoid taking opioids because she is afraid of getting addicted. She has had many spinal injections. She presented at a pain clinic with a complaint of low back pain. Her pain level ranges from 0 to 10 and increases with activities. Patient's pain medications include acetaminophen, diazepam and lidocaine gel. She is cognitively intact and denies any history of alcohol use or any psychiatric disorders.

Treatment: the patient was continued on Tylenol extra strength, muscle relaxer, and topical medications and imaging studies were ordered.

QUESTIONS:

Type of Pain Acute/ Chronic: _____ *Duration of Pain* _____

Psychosocial Comorbidities _____

Cognitive Impairment _____

Opioids Medications _____

Length of Time on Opioids Medications _____

Prior Treatments Received for the
Condition _____

Providers Pain management _____
Psychiatrist/Behavioral/Addiction _____

Psychosocial /financial Support _____

Others _____

ANSWER - CASE # THREE

Class _____2_____ **Group** _____A_____

FOCAS: 2A.

Comments: This case is pretty straightforward, an elderly patient with no documented history of opioids. She has chronic pain which is treated with none opioid medications and procedures.

The patient's group classification would change if she starts on opioid; this would be changed to **Group 2B**.

CASE # FOUR

This is a 51-year-old female who presents for initial evaluation for left knee pain as well as low back pain. She sustained a work-related injury almost two years ago which resulted in her having back surgery. Type of surgery was unknown at the time of her presentation. However, the patient improved after surgery. She has been on and off of opioids medications and was referred by her primary care provider for pain management.

She denies any illicit drug use, she has a history of depression and is being treated with Paxil for several years. There are no known cognitive deficits.

Treatment: she was started on tramadol, a muscle relaxer, and anti-inflammatory.

QUESTIONS:

Type of Pain Acute/ Chronic: _____ *Duration of Pain* _____

Psychosocial Comorbidities _____

Cognitive Impairment _____

Opioids Medications _____

Length of Time on Opioids Medications _____

Prior Treatments Received for the
Condition _____

Providers Pain management _____
Psychiatrist/Behavioral/Addiction _____

Psychosocial /financial Support _____

Others _____

ANSWER - CASE # FOUR

Class _____3_____ Group _____C_____

FOCAS: 3C

Comments: This patient might have been in **Group 2C**, probably got well with occasional use of opioids and other medications to help control her pain. However, the patient is now a chronic pain patient requiring more involved care and management of her pain.

If the patient had no psychiatric disorder or other comorbidities such as cognitive impairment, substance abuse – none opioids, then she would be placed in **Group 3B.**

CASE # FIVE

Patient JN is a 66-year-old male who has a diagnosis of rheumatoid arthritis and osteoarthritis. A pain management clinic has followed him for over six years he has been maintained on fentanyl patch 25 µg as well as Percocet 10/325 mg three times a day as needed. He also is treated periodically with spinal injections as well as joint injections to help control his pain.

The patient denies any history of non-opioid substance abuse, psychiatric or cognitive disorder; he follows up with his pain management physician as well as his primary care and a rheumatologist as required.

Treatment: fentanyl, Percocet, other none narcotics – Lyrica, Zanaflex.

QUESTIONS:

Type of Pain Acute/ Chronic: _____ *Duration of Pain* _____

Psychosocial Comorbidities _____

Cognitive Impairment _____

Opioids Medications _____

Length of Time on Opioids Medications _____

Prior Treatments Received for the
Condition _____

Providers Pain management _____
Psychiatrist/Behavioral/Addiction _____

Psychosocial /financial Support _____

Others _____

ANSWER - CASE # FIVE

Class _____4_____ Group _____A_____

FOCAS:4A

Comments: This case is pretty straight forward. The patient is being manage in a pain management clinic. His pain appears to be appropriately controlled with medications and procedures.

CASE # SIX

Patient PC is a 78-year-old female with complaint of bilateral hips pain, back pain, shoulder and knee pain. She has been in pain management for over five years, her pain level range at about 8 to 10 out of 10 while currently on Percocet 10/326 mg four times a day, morphine sulfate 30 mg twice a day, Lyrica some 75 mg twice a day and Zanaflex 2 mg twice a day. She was seen in consultation by an orthopedic surgeon for her knees and hips. She also has periodic spinal injection as well as joint injections with some improvement however not sustained.

She's been followed by psychiatry for depression and anxiety and is treated with BuSpar, trazodone, risperidone, and Lexapro. She denies any use of non-opioid substance abuse and has no cognitive deficits.

Treatment: as indicated above

QUESTIONS:

Type of Pain Acute/ Chronic: _____*Duration of Pain*_____

*Psychosocial Comorbidities*_____

*Cognitive Impairment*_____

*Opioids Medications*_____

*Length of Time on Opioids Medications*_____

Prior Treatments Received for the
*Condition*_____

*Providers Pain management*_____
Psychiatrist/Behavioral/Addiction _____

*Psychosocial /financial Support*_____

*Others*_____

ANSWER - CASE # SIX

Class _____4_____ Group _____C_____

FOCAS: 4C

Comments: this patient has significant comorbidities and significant pain related symptoms. Also has significant psychiatric comorbidities which are being treated. In spite of her treatment she is not well and has unsatisfactory level of pain control.

This patient would have been classified as belonging to **Group 4B** if she had no psychiatric illness or other relevant comorbidities.

CASE # SEVEN

Patient MD is a 63-year-old female who was involved in a motor vehicle accident about 14 months ago, she complained of low back pain and neck pain. She was treated with Tylenol, Percocet 5/325 mg TID PRN, Flexeril 5 mg bid and Gabapentin 300 mg QHS. She stated that her pain varies from 4 to 9 out of 10 and is associated with radiation to the lower extremities. The patient underwent epidural steroid injections for low back pain and continued with her current medications with gradual tapering. She did well and was referred for physical therapy for 6 to 8 weeks and currently takes none opioid medication occasionally.

She denies any history of non-opioid substance abuse, denies any psychiatric illness and has no cognitive deficits.

Treatment: as above.

QUESTIONS:

Type of Pain Acute/ Chronic: _____ *Duration of Pain*_____

*Psychosocial Comorbidities*_____

*Cognitive Impairment*_____

*Opioids Medications*_____

*Length of Time on Opioids Medications*_____

*Prior Treatments Received for the
Condition*_____

*Providers Pain management*_____
Psychiatrist/Behavioral/Addiction _____

*Psychosocial /financial Support*_____

*Others*_____

ANSWER - CASE # SEVEN

Class _____3_____ Group _____A_____

FOCAS: 3A

Comments: This case is also reasonably straight forward, the patient was treated for chronic pain, was seen in consultation by a pain physician and did well.

This patient would have been classified as belonging to **Group 3B** if she had failed to respond to treatment and continued with escalating opioid medications.

CASE # EIGHT

Patient SZ is a 56-year-old female who has a history of low back pain and headaches, she has been in pain management for about 4- 5 years and is currently being treated with fentanyl 25 μg as well as Percocet 10/325 mg three times a day, gabapentin, baclofen, Fioricet, ibuprofen, and lidocaine ointment. She has had multiple procedures for low back pain and had modest improvements of for pain. She at times has overtaken her opioids medications and had one prescription filled from another doctor for opioids.

She's been followed by a psychiatrist as well as psychologists; she is on Wellbutrin XL, Buspirone, Valium, and Cymbalta. She has no cognitive deficits; she has good psychosocial support.

Treatment: as above.

QUESTIONS:

Type of Pain Acute/ Chronic: _____ *Duration of Pain* _____

Psychosocial Comorbidities _____

Cognitive Impairment _____

Opioids Medications _____

Length of Time on Opioids Medications _____

Prior Treatments Received for the
Condition _____

Providers Pain management _____
Psychiatrist/Behavioral/Addiction _____

Psychosocial /financial Support _____

Others _____

ANSWER - CASE # EIGHT

Class _____4_____ Group _____C_____

FOCAS: 4C

Comments: This case is more complex. However, the classification is appropriate, although her pain and overall condition have improved with the treatment she is still not well. In addition, the level of support required to maintain her is significant. She is bordering on belonging to **Group 5A**; she is not addicted but probably has developed tolerance or opioid dependence. Without appropriate treatment, this patient may become an opioid use disorder patient.

CASE # NINE

DS is a 50-year-old male who has a long history of low back pain related to a job injury sustained many years ago. He has been on high-dose opioids and has been in and out of pain clinics, some of which he was discharged from. His last clinic was a Suboxone clinic where he was discharged after testing positive for marijuana. He stated that his pain ranges from 7 to 10 with radiation to both lower extremities. He further stated that he is using heroin to help control his withdrawal. He said that it costs approximately $30-$40 for each dose purchased. He presents to a pain clinic for treatment of Suboxone his urine confirmation test was positive for heroin, fentanyl, morphine, and oxycodone.

He stated that he lives alone, all of his family members live in another state. He stated that he attends church and has an active church family. He admitted to using illegal drugs as described above as well as prior history of cocaine use.

He also has a history of anxiety and depression, denies any significant alcohol use. In addition, he has significant cardiac and pulmonary diseases.

Treatment: after complete assessments – Suboxone

QUESTIONS:

Type of Pain Acute/ Chronic: _____ *Duration of Pain* _____

Psychosocial Comorbidities _____

Cognitive Impairment _____

Opioids Medications _____

Length of Time on Opioids Medications _____

Prior Treatments Received for the
Condition _____

Providers Pain management _____
Psychiatrist/Behavioral/Addiction _____

Psychosocial /financial Support _____

Others _____

ANSWER - CASE # NINE

Class _____5_____ Group _____C_____

FOCAS: 5C

Comments: This case is significant for several reasons; the patient is still actively using illicit drugs, he has significant comorbidities (cardiac/pulmonary) and has poor psychosocial support. Because of these factors in part, he is an extremely high-risk patient for administering any treatment. However, if he is not treated, this is the type of patient that is most likely to die from heroin laced with illicitly manufactured fentanyl or simply from any of the illicit drugs and or combination of them.

Consider the scenario where this patient has good psychosocial support, no cognitive or psychiatric disorders, and no use of **illicit non-opioid drugs,** but simply failed management of his pain on prescription opioids, and then possible resort to abusing illegal opioids. The most appropriate classification would be classified as belonging **Group 5A** (Probably hypothetically was a **Group 4B** patient before), now addicted to opioids.

This patient may also have been classified in **Group 5XB** before being addicted and now in **Group 5A.**

Group 5B, also an opioid addiction group would be applicable for patients who have somewhat moderate psychosocial support but has no significant history of nonopioids illicit drug abuse, as well as no psychiatric or cognitive disorders. So, this group is the intermediate group between the more extreme addiction **Group 5C** and less complex addiction **Group 5A.** Therefore, one, for example, would expect to see a more significant history of illegal drug abuse of opioids associated with those patients classified as belonging to **Group 5B** than **Group 5A** and even more abuse with **Group 5C.**

CASE # TEN

BJ is a 16-year-old high school male student who presented at the school nurse with his father who wanted to discuss some changes that he has noticed in his son behavior and overall actions. His son denies using any illicit drugs. However, he consented to have a urine drug test which was positive for opioids. When confronted with this BJ admitted to taking pills from his mother's medicine cabinet in which he said he does every now and again. BJ's mother is on chronic opioid for low back pain; she had a related car accident several years ago.

BJ otherwise have no other drug history, has no pain or any complaint of any health problems, he has no cognitive deficits. He is considered to be a normal regular student.

Treatment: counseling

QUESTIONS:

Type of Pain Acute/ Chronic: _____ *Duration of Pain*_____

*Psychosocial Comorbidities*_____

*Cognitive Impairment*_____

*Opioids Medications*_____

*Length of Time on Opioids Medications*_____

*Prior Treatments Received for the Condition*_____

*Providers Pain management*_____
Psychiatrist/Behavioral/Addiction _____

*Psychosocial /financial Support*_____

*Others*_____

ANSWER - CASE # TEN

Class _____5_____ Group _____XA_____

FOCAS: 5XA.

Comments: all that we know is what BJ said, we don't know how accurate that is. We also know that BJ has no pain or no other comorbidities, therefore, the classification would be as indicated.

If BJ had pain and had no other comorbidities such as psychiatric disorder, behavioral disorder, cognitive disorder or non-opioids substance abuse disorder, then he would be classified as belonging to **Group 5XB**.

Similarity, if BJ had pain or no pain and had any of the comorbidities indicated above you would be classified as belonging to **Group 5XC**.

CASE # ELEVEN

Mr. JT operates a convenience store, a restaurant and is the owner of a large warehouse that he receives and ships out various products. Among the products that he ships out and receives are heroin and illicitly manufactured fentanyl. Although he knows what is in these containers he never himself directly handle these drugs. He has key personnel that knows where to send and whom to send them to.

Mr. JT has no medical problems, no cognitive deficits, and no psychiatric illness. he is considered to be in good standing in the society.

Treatment: none

QUESTIONS:

Type of Pain Acute/ Chronic: _____*Duration of Pain*_____

*Psychosocial Comorbidities*_____

*Cognitive Impairment*_____

*Opioids Medications*_____

*Length of Time on Opioids Medications*_____

*Prior Treatments Received for the
Condition*_____

*Providers Pain management*_____
Psychiatrist/Behavioral/Addiction _____

*Psychosocial /financial Support*_____

*Others*_____

ANSWER - CASE # ELEVEN

Class _____5___ Group ____XD or XS_____

FOCAS: 5XD or 5XS.

Comments: Mr. JT and his crew are classified as a dealer and or supplier; his supplies may be coming from local or foreign.

CASE # TWELVE

Ms. CT is a 56-year-old female that has been followed by a pain clinic for the past for years; she has neck pain, low back pain, as well as pain involving both hands. She is status post back surgery times two, last one approximately 6 – 7 years ago. She has been maintained on Oxycodone 20 mg three times a day and morphine sulfate 30 mg twice a day, also Flexeril 10 mg three times a day, gabapentin 900 mg three times a day, and lidocaine ointment 5% for three times a day. She's also been seen and followed by psychiatry, she is on Cymbalta 60 mg daily, as well as Xanax 0.5 mg twice a day as needed.

Her social history is significant for the history of smoking one pack of cigarettes per day, history of cocaine and marijuana use in the past. She is married, however, has been on disability for approximately ten years. She has adequate healthcare coverage.

Treatment: she was treated as above. However, she was found to have positive marijuana and cocaine in her urine as well as receiving multiple opioid prescriptions from other providers. She was discharged from the pain practice for which she had been seen for several years. In addition to her illegal drugs patient was warned several times for overtaking medications and have use opioid prescription from other physicians at least twice in the past.

After she was discharged, the patient had difficulty finding another pain clinic and resorted to buying opioids and other drugs in the street. She continued to buy drugs on the street and was seen in consultation after being admitted to a medical unit for an overdose of opioids.

Treatment: as above

QUESTIONS:

Type of Pain Acute/ Chronic: _____ *Duration of Pain* _____

Psychosocial Comorbidities _____

Cognitive Impairment _____

Opioids Medications _____

Length of Time on Opioids Medications _____

Prior Treatments Received for the
*Condition*_____

*Providers Pain management*_____
Psychiatrist/Behavioral/Addiction _____

*Psychosocial /financial Support*_____

*Others*_____

ANSWER- CASE # TWELVE

Class _____5_____ Group _____XC_____

FOCAS: 5XC.

Comments: The patient probably would've been classified as a member of the **Group 4C**, however once discharged and resorting to illicit drugs without supervision and overdosing all these factors more than meet the requirements for **Group 5 XC**.

If the above patient had none of the psychosocial/drug-related issues or psychiatric disorder and had pain and was discharged for overtaking medications are abusing medication while in a pain clinic, then the classification would have been **Group 5XB**.

CASE # THIRTEEN

Patient RJ 21-year-old female who was taken by her mother to see her primary care doctor because she believes that her daughter had lost interest in her activities of daily living, her hygiene and mental status have appeared to have declined. RJ had been living with her parents since birth and is considered to be developmentally delayed. She attended a special needs school from which she graduated. Her mother stated that she has been dating. She believes that her new boyfriend is very helpful and have been very kind to her. The patient is an Adderall and birth control medication. She denies any illicit drugs or alcohol use.

Treatment: a primary care physician ordered the urine toxicology tests which was significant for methamphetamine as well as opioids and marijuana. RJ stated that she doesn't do any drugs.

QUESTIONS:

Type of Pain Acute/ Chronic: _____ *Duration of Pain*_____

*Psychosocial Comorbidities*_____

*Cognitive Impairment*_____

*Opioids Medications*_____

*Length of Time on Opioids Medications*_____

*Prior Treatments Received for the Condition*_____

*Providers Pain management*_____
Psychiatrist/Behavioral/Addiction _____

*Psychosocial /financial Support*_____

*Others*_____

ANSWER - CASE # THIRTEEN

Class _____5_____ Group _____XC_____

FOCAS: 5XC.

Comments: this is pretty straightforward, because of patient cognitive impairment and opioid use any illicit drugs should be classified into this group.

Similarly, even if she had only been taking opioid illegally, she would still be classified in this group. Also, whether or not she has pain, this would be this group of her classification.

On the other hand, if the patient were a 21-year-old female with pain from whatever cause, with no developmental delay, illicit drug use other than opioids and no psychiatric disorders/ disorder then her classification would've been **Group 5XB**.

CASE # FOURTEEN

JL is a 25-year-old female who went to see her pastor/Bishop for confession. She stated that she felt guilty about using heroin and some other stuff, but she is not sure what they were. She said that she was with her boyfriend who works for the fire department in her community. She is not quite sure what to do, but she indicated that she doesn't want to get hooked on any drugs.

She seemed very frantic and anxious; she stated that she had never done drugs before and she doesn't want her family to know. She doesn't want to go to a counseling center because she is afraid that she will see drug addicts there.

She has no cognitive deficits or psychiatric disorder, no significant pain or other medical condition and has excellent family support. She further stated that she is madly in love with her boyfriend.

Treatment: the pastor tried to arrange a meeting with her family members, but she was having none of that instead she walked away.

QUESTIONS:

Type of Pain Acute/ Chronic: _____ *Duration of Pain* _____

Psychosocial Comorbidities _____

Cognitive Impairment _____

Opioids Medications _____

Length of Time on Opioids Medications _____

Prior Treatments Received for the
Condition _____

Providers Pain management _____
Psychiatrist/Behavioral/Addiction _____

Psychosocial /financial Support _____

Others _____

ANSWER - CASE # FOURTEEN

Class _____5_____ Group _____XA_____

FOCAS: 5XA.

Comments: this is also fairly straightforward, although her drug use seems to be very early at this stage, one can never be sure what extent she is truthful. Also, it's unknown at this stage what she actually took regarding illegal drugs.

CASE # FIFTEEN

Mr. XY was seen and evaluated for the first time today in a pain clinic and have complained of low back pain and right calcaneus fracture for which he has surgeries. He stated that his back pain is at a tolerable level about the 4 to 5 out of 10 for about three years. However, his foot pain is related to the calcaneus fracture varies in pain from 0/10 to 10/10. He is S/P surgery five years ago, and only use topical creams, anti-inflammatory, and modification of his shoes. He has no opioids use for four years.

He also stated that he was previously treated for bipolar disorder in the past but is currently not on any medication and is doing fine, and has not seen a psychiatrist for about 12 years. He is cognitively intact, denies any use of illicit drugs except for marijuana which is used in the distant past. He has good family support, he works as a manager at a major company and is married with children.

Treatment: continue topical pain medication, anti-inflammatory, tramadol, and gabapentin.

QUESTIONS:

Type of Pain Acute/ Chronic: _____ *Duration of Pain* _____

Psychosocial Comorbidities _____

Cognitive Impairment _____

Opioids Medications _____

Length of Time on Opioids Medications _____

Prior Treatments Received for the
Condition _____

Providers Pain management _____
Psychiatrist/Behavioral/Addiction _____

Psychosocial /financial Support _____

Others _____

ANSWER - CASE # FIFTEEN

Class _____3_____ Group _____C_____

FOCAS:3C

Comments: This case is a little more interesting and probably little more challenging, it is very likely that at the time when patient pain had subsided to the point where he stopped using opioids that his **Group** was **3C**. This is still reasonable to start is the treatment.

However, this patient could've continued on non-opioids however, that is likely not to be adequate as he has been doing that for several years without significant improvement. Reassessment of his ankle/foot injuries may enable potential alternative treatment that might improve his overall pain. His back pain will require full evaluation to determine the cause and possible treatment options other than opioids.

Group 4C involves primarily patient what had extensive opioid treatment and consultation/intervention for management of their pain. This did not apply in this case. Also, **Groups 4B and 3B** would not be appropriate because of the patient's psychiatric history and illegal drug use, although remote they should still be considered as significant factors.

Clearly not every case will fit perfectly in each group.

CASE # SIXTEEN

Mr. ST is an is-60-year-old male who was diagnosed with low back pain. He also has a history of multiple sclerosis without any significant recent exacerbation. He has been attending a pain clinic for more than four years but has been transferred to a new clinic after being discharged from three other clinics. He is currently taking fentanyl 25 µg patch, Percocet 10/325 one tablet four times a day as needed, gabapentin 400 mg three times a day.

He has had occasional spinal injections/joints injections to help control his pain. However, he continues to run out of his medications sometimes as much as one week ahead of his scheduled visit. He has had multiple inconsistent urine drug tests and was discharged from the new facility. He resorted to purchasing medications on the street and was recently arrested for trafficking prescription drugs.

He denies any history of illegal drugs uses, has no cognitive or psychiatric deficits/disorder. He lives with his wife. He is on disability for 15 years.

Treatment: as above

QUESTIONS:

Type of Pain Acute/ Chronic: _____ *Duration of Pain* _____

Psychosocial Comorbidities _____

Cognitive Impairment _____

Opioids Medications _____

Length of Time on Opioids Medications _____

Prior Treatments Received for the
Condition _____

Providers Pain management _____
Psychiatrist/Behavioral/Addiction _____

Psychosocial /financial Support _____

Others _____

ANSWER- CASE # SIXTEEN

Class _____5_____ Group _____XB_____

FOCAS:5XB.

Comments: This is relatively straightforward, the patient who was managed in a pain management facility, however, was discharged because of noncompliance and probably demonstrating tolerance or opioid dependence and was discharged for overtaking opioids medications. He subsequently started using illegal prescription medications and illicit opioids. However, with a history of pain and treatment and subsequent use of illicit drugs is classification is appropriate.

CASE # SEVENTEEN

JB is a 23-year-old female who is in her second year of college; she has finished the first year with some struggle. In her second year, she is having academic issues which she attributed to; difficulty staying awake and feels tired. She has been taking some pills from a friend who told her that they would help her, she does not know what they were. She was at a party and was given something in a drink and told that it was Ecstasy MDS. She woke up in an emergency room and can only remember what happened prior to consuming her drink.

She remained in the hospital on a behavioral unit; she was tested positive for opioids, marijuana and Ecstasy MDS from a urine sample taken in the emergency room. Her physical examination was also significant for what was described as an apparent sexual assault. She now has some confusion along with memory issues and difficulty processing things that are considered simple and routine.

Treatment......?

QUESTIONS:

Type of Pain Acute/ Chronic: _____ *Duration of Pain* _____

Psychosocial Comorbidities _____

Cognitive Impairment _____

Opioids Medications _____

Length of Time on Opioids Medications _____

Prior Treatments Received for the
Condition _____

Providers Pain management _____
Psychiatrist/Behavioral/Addiction _____

Psychosocial /financial Support _____

Others _____

ANSWER - CASE # SEVENTEEN

Class _____5_____ Group _____XC_____

FOCAS: 5XC

Comments: This is somewhat straightforward. She has no apparent prior comorbidities but has a history of substance abuse or use, although it's unclear what she was taken or given prior to her hospitalization. It is possible that she may have been taken an herbal supplement or other natural products that are legal, however, since this is unknown the XC category is more appropriate. Moreover, she was tested positive for marijuana and opioids.

If she had no significant substance abuse or psychiatric illness, cognitive issues without pain, this would place her in **Group 5XA**, or in **Group 5XB** if she was being treated for pain but has no psychiatric or substance abuse issues, etc.

CASE # EIGHTEEN

JT is that 22-year-old female who was walking down the street and slip and sprain her right ankle. She stated that her pain level is 9 to 10 out of 10. She has never been in used any opioid and is not in any other medications.

She attends college, has no cognitive or psychiatric disorder and denies any illicit drug use.

Treatment......?

QUESTIONS:

Type of Pain Acute/ Chronic: _____ *Duration of Pain* _____

Psychosocial Comorbidities _____

Cognitive Impairment _____

Opioids Medications _____

Length of Time on Opioids Medications _____

Prior Treatments Received for the
Condition _____

Providers Pain management _____
Psychiatrist/Behavioral/Addiction _____

Psychosocial /financial Support _____

Others _____

ANSWER- CASE # EIGHTEEN

Class _____1_____ Group _____A_OR B_____

FOCAS :1A or 1B.

Comments: This is straightforward. JT group classification will depend on what medication she is started on.

If she started on non-opioids, then she is in **Group 1A**. If she started on an opioid, she is in **Group 1B**.

She is, of course, started at **Class 0, Group 0.**

CASE # NINETEEN

Mr. RT is an 89-year-old male who was walking and sustained a fall since then has been complaining of back pain for about one week; he was seen in the emergency room at the hospital and had x-rays which were negative. He is also had chronic pain involving his joins and back pain before his fall, however; he was not taking any medications. He stated that he has been in pain for several years. He sometimes forgets things; he was seen by a neurologist who thinks he may have an early sign of dementia, however, is okay to live alone.

He has no history of psychiatric disorder or history of illegal of drug use.

Treatment......?

QUESTIONS:

Type of Pain Acute/ Chronic: _____ *Duration of Pain*_____

*Psychosocial Comorbidities*_____

*Cognitive Impairment*_____

*Opioids Medications*_____

*Length of Time on Opioids Medications*_____

Prior Treatments Received for the
*Condition*_____

*Providers Pain management*_____
Psychiatrist/Behavioral/Addiction _____

*Psychosocial /financial Support*_____

*Others*_____

ANSWER - CASE # NINETEEN

Class _____2_____ Group _____A_ or B_____

FOCAS: 2A or 2B.

 Comments: This is straightforward. RT group classification will depend on what medication he is started on.

If he started on a non-opioid, then he is in **Group 2A**. If he started on opioid, he is in **Group 2B.**

CASE # TWENTY

Mr. TD is well-known as a drug dealer in the area, he was involved in a motor vehicle accident and was seen in a pain clinic and treated for low back pain and neck pain. He then had physical therapy and was discharged home with pain medications along with anti-inflammatory and muscle relaxers to continue taking.

He denies any psychiatric disorder/cognitive disorder. He does admit dealing in illegal drugs and opioids.

Treatment: as above

QUESTIONS:

Type of Pain Acute/ Chronic: _____ *Duration of Pain*_____

*Psychosocial Comorbidities*_____

*Cognitive Impairment*_____

*Opioids Medications*_____

*Length of Time on Opioids Medications*_____

Prior Treatments Received for the
*Condition*_____

*Providers Pain management*_____
Psychiatrist/Behavioral/Addiction _____

*Psychosocial /financial Support*_____

*Others*_____

ANSWER CASE # TWENTY

Class _____5_____ Group _____XDB_____

FOCAS: 5XDB.

Comments: This is the case where a drug dealer with pain is receiving treatment or using opioids illegally.

If this were a supplier, the classification would be **Group 5XSB.**

Also, if a drug dealer or supplier had psychiatric, cognitive or substance use issue that is non-opioid and were using opioids, (with or without pain), the group classification would be **Group 5XDC or 5XSC** respectively.

Without any comorbidities than the classification would be **Group 5XDA or 5XSA** respectively.

CHAPTER THREE

Useful Tools for Assessment and Evaluation of Patients on Opioids

Calculating Morphine Milligram Equivalents (MME)

How to calculate Morphine **Milligrams Equivalent (MME)** daily dose also called **Morphine Equivalent Dose (MED)** daily or **Morphine Equivalent Daily (MED)** Dose. The calculations of MME use morphine as the reference opioid base on the strength or potency of other opioids. There are many different types of methods and or applications that are available for calculations. There are therefore different results that are obtained sometimes depending on the applications or methods that are used. So be aware of the applications that you can install on your smartphone or tablets, as well as the various computer programs that are available and make sure that whatever you use reconciled with some known standard.

Calculating Morphine Milligram Equivalents (MME)	
OPIOID (doses in mg/day except where noted)	**CONVERSION FACTOR**
Codeine	0.15
Fentanyl transdermal (in mcg/hr.)	2.4
Hydrocodone	1
Hydromorphone	4
Methadone	
1-20 mg/day	4
21-40 mg/day	8
41-60 g/day	10
$\geq 61 - 80$ mg/day	12
Morphine	1
Oxycodone	1.5
Oxymorphone	3

These dose conversions are estimated and cannot account for all individual differences in genetics and pharmacokinetics. (CDC protocol).

1. **Determine** the total daily amount of each opioid the patient takes
2. **Convert** each to MMEs—multiply the dose for each opioid by the conversion factor.
3. **Add** them together.

The CDC has a conversion table which is available for use. Although it does not cover some opioids, it still forms a significant reference point from which to determine the MME of each patient that are prescribed opioids. The table and the conversion factors are shown above.

Methadone and Fentanyl seem to vary in the results calculated in a number of different programs.

Buprenorphine a partial agonist is not included in the CDC calculations, most calculations are done with a conversion factor of **1.8** (for each daily microgram unit).

Tramadol a conversion factor of **0.1**

Reference

Centers for Disease Control and Prevention.
https://www.cdc.gov/drugoverdose/pdf/calculating_total_dose-a.pdf Accessed May 30, 2018.

DEA DRUGS (CONTROLLED SUBSTANCES) CLASSIFICATION SCHEDULE I-V

This section included a table showing how drugs are generally classified by the Drug Enforcement Administration(**DEA**).

CLASS	CRITERIA	EXAMPLES OF DRUGS
Schedule I	No currently accepted medical use and a high potential for abuse.	Some examples of Schedule I drugs are: heroin, lysergic acid diethylamide (LSD), marijuana (cannabis), 3,4-methylenedioxymethamphetamine (ecstasy), methaqualone, and peyote
Schedule II	High potential for abuse, with use potentially leading to severe psychological or physical dependence. These drugs are also considered dangerous	Combination products with less than 15 milligrams of hydrocodone per dosage unit (Vicodin), cocaine, methamphetamine, methadone, hydromorphone (Dilaudid), meperidine (Demerol), oxycodone (OxyContin), fentanyl, Dexedrine, Adderall, and Ritalin
Schedule III	Moderate to low potential for physical and psychological dependence. Schedule III drugs abuse potential is less than Schedule I and Schedule II drugs but more than Schedule IV	Products containing less than 90 milligrams of codeine per dosage unit (Tylenol with codeine), ketamine, anabolic steroids, testosterone

Schedule IV	Low potential for abuse and low risk of dependence	Xanax, Soma, Darvon, Darvocet, Valium, Ativan, Talwin, Ambien, Tramadol
Schedule V	Lower potential for abuse than Schedule IV and consists of preparations containing limited quantities of certain narcotics. Schedule V drugs are generally used for antidiarrheal, antitussive, and analgesic purposes.	Cough preparations with less than 200 milligrams of codeine or per 100 milliliters (Robitussin AC), Lomotil, Motofen, Lyrica, Parepectolin

This also is very useful in your understanding of the potential danger and usefulness of some of these substances/drugs.

The Controlled Substance Act of 1970 in part empowered the DEA to classify drugs/control substances. The drugs/substances are classified as indicated in the table above into five classes or schedules depending upon the substance/drug's acceptable medical use and their potential for abuse or to cause dependence. Drugs or substances can be added, or class/schedule changed depending on the current or new information.

CDC 2016 SUMMARY GUIDELINE FOR CHRONIC PAIN
GUIDELINE FOR PRESCRIBING OPIOIDS FOR CHRONIC PAIN

IMPROVING PRACTICE THROUGH RECOMMENDATIONS

CDC's Guideline for Prescribing Opioids for Chronic Pain is intended to improve communication between providers and patients about the risks and benefits of opioid therapy for chronic pain, improve the safety and effectiveness of pain treatment, and reduce the risks associated with long-term opioid therapy, including opioid use disorder and overdose. The Guideline is not intended for patients who are in active cancer treatment, palliative care, or end-of-life care.

DETERMINING WHEN TO INITIATE OR CONTINUE OPIOIDS FOR CHRONIC PAIN

- Nonpharmacologic therapy and nonopioid pharmacologic therapy are preferred for chronic pain. Clinicians should consider opioid therapy only if expected benefits for both pain and function are anticipated to outweigh risks to the patient. If opioids are used, they should be combined with nonpharmacologic therapy and nonopioid pharmacologic therapy, as appropriate.
- Before starting opioid therapy for chronic pain, clinicians should establish treatment goals with all patients, including realistic goals for pain and function, and should consider how opioid therapy will be discontinued if benefits do not outweigh risks. Clinicians should continue opioid therapy only if there is clinically meaningful improvement in pain and function that outweighs risks to patient safety.
- Before starting and periodically during opioid therapy, clinicians should discuss with patients known risks and realistic benefits of opioid therapy and patient and clinician responsibilities for managing therapy.

CLINICAL REMINDERS

- Opioids are not first-line or routine therapy for chronic pain
- Establish and measure goals for pain and function
- Discuss benefits and risks and availability of non-opioid therapies with patient.

OPIOID SELECTION, DOSAGE, DURATION, FOLLOW-UP, AND DISCONTINUATION

- When starting opioid therapy for chronic pain, clinicians should prescribe immediate-release opioids instead of extended-release/long-acting (ER/ LA) opioids.

- When opioids are started, clinicians should prescribe the lowest effective dosage. Clinicians should use caution when prescribing opioids at any dosage, should carefully reassess evidence of individual benefits and risks when considering increasing dosage to ≥50 morphine milligram equivalents (MME)/day, and should avoid increasing dosage to ≥90 MME/day or carefully justify a decision to titrate dosage to ≥90 MME/day.

- Long-term opioid use often begins with treatment of acute pain. When opioids are used for acute pain, clinicians should prescribe the lowest effective dose of immediate-release opioids and should prescribe no greater quantity than needed for the expected duration of pain severe enough to require opioids. Three days or less will often be sufficient; more than seven days will rarely be needed. Clinicians should evaluate benefits and harms with patients within 1 to 4 weeks of starting opioid therapy for chronic pain or of dose escalation.

- Clinicians should evaluate benefits and harms of continued therapy with patients every 3 months or more frequently. If benefits do not outweigh harms of continued opioid therapy, clinicians should optimize other therapies and work with patients to taper opioids to lower dosages or to taper and discontinue opioids.

CLINICAL REMINDERS

- Use immediate-release opioids when starting
- Start low and go slow
- When opioids are needed for acute pain, prescribe no more than needed
- Do not prescribe ER/LA opioids for acute pain
- Follow-up and re-evaluate risk of harm; reduce dose or taper and discontinue if needed.

ASSESSING RISK ANDADDRESSING HARMS OF OPIOID USE

- Before starting and periodically during continuation of opioid therapy, clinicians should evaluate risk factors for opioid-related harms. Clinicians should incorporate into the management plan strategies to mitigate risk, including considering offering naloxone when factors that increase risk for opioid overdose, such as history of overdose, history of substance use disorder, higher opioid dosages ($\geq$50 MME/day), or concurrent benzodiazepine use, are present.
- Clinicians should review the patient's history of controlled substance prescriptions using state prescription drug monitoring program (PDMP) data to determine whether the patient is receiving opioid dosages or dangerous combinations that put him or her at high risk for overdose. Clinicians should review PDMP data when starting opioid therapy for chronic pain and periodically during opioid therapy for chronic pain, ranging from every prescription to every 3 months.
- When prescribing opioids for chronic pain, clinicians should use urine drug testing before starting opioid therapy and consider urine drug testing at least annually to assess for prescribed medications as well as other controlled prescription drugs and illicit drugs.
- Clinicians should avoid prescribing opioid pain medication and benzodiazepines concurrently whenever possible.
- Clinicians should offer or arrange evidence-based treatment (usually medication-assisted treatment with buprenorphine or methadone in combination with behavioral therapies) for patients with opioid use disorder.

CLINICAL REMINDERS

Evaluate risk factors for opioid-related harms
- Check PDMP for high dosages and prescriptions from other providers
- Use urine drug testing to identify prescribed substances and undisclosed use
- Avoid concurrent benzodiazepine and opioid prescribing
- Arrange treatment for opioid use disorder if needed

LEARN MORE | www.cdc.gov/drugoverdose/prescribing/guideline.html

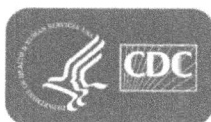

**U.S. Department of
Health and Human Services**
Centers for Disease
Control and Prevention

Table of Different Drug Classes, Street Names, Generic Names, Route of Ingestion, Appearance, and Schedule.

Tables of different drug classes ranging from opioids, central nervous system depressants, central nervous system stimulants, hallucinogens, psychoactive drugs and substances that are commonly abuse or have the potential for abuse or misuse.

This is intended used primarily as a reference and also will be helpful to you in understanding and appreciating the different types of drugs/substances that are available. This is of course only a partial list of the numerous compounds that are available. So, familiarize yourself with them and some of the different street names that are associated with these drugs.

PRESCRIPTION OPIOIDS					
NARCOTICS	**TRADE NAMES**	**STREET NAMES**	**APPEARANCES**	**ROUTE OF INGESTION**	**SCHEDULE**
Buprenorphine	Suboxone, Buprenex, and Subutex,	Bupe	Tablets	Swallowed, skin patch, injected	III
Codeine	Codeine (various brand names)	Captain Cody, Cody, Lean, Schoolboy, Sizzurp, Purple Drank.	Tablet, capsule, liquid	Injected, swallowed (often mixed with soda and flavorings)	IV
Fentanyl	Duragesic, Actiq, Fentora, Sublimaze	China White, Dance Fever Lollipop, Perc-O-Pop, China White, Mexican Brown Apache, China Girl, Friend, Goodfella, Jackpot, Murder 8, Tango and Cash, TNT	Crushed, cake-like, crumbly, powdered, patch tablets, film, buccal tablets	Swallowed, injected, skin patch snorted	II
Heroine (Not prescribed in the US)	No commercial name	Brown sugar, China White, Dope, H, Horse, Junk, Skag, Skink, Smack, White Horse	White or brownish powder or black sticky substance is known as "black tar heroin	Smoked, snorted, injected	I
Hydrocodone	Vicodin, Vicoprofen, Reprexain, Ibudone	Vikes, Codone, Hydro, Viko, Norco, Watson-387	Tablets, capsules, liquid	Swallowed snorted, injected	II
Hydromorphone	Dilaudid	Footballs, Juice, Dillies, smak	Liquid, suppository, tablets	Ingested, rectal, swallowed, snorted	II
Meperidine	Demerol	Demmies, Pain Killer	White crystalline substance, liquid, tablets	Snorted, Oral, injected	II
Methadone	Dolophine, Methadose	Dollie, Amidone, Fizzies, With MDMA: Chocolate Chip Cookies	Tablets, solution	Swallowed, snorted, injected	II

Morphine (M), Morphine Sulfate	MS Contin, Duramorph,	M, Miss Emma, Atom Bomb, Monkey, White Stuff	White powder or crystals, clear liquid, tablets, capsules, suppository	Swallowed, nasal, smoked, injected	II
Oxycodone	Roxicodone, Roxicef, OxyContin, Percocan, Percocet	O, C., Roxi, Molly, Perk, Oxycet, Oxycotton, Oxy, Hillbilly Heroin, Percs	White to off-white powder, as tablets, liquid, capsule	Swallowed Chewed, snorted, injected	II
Oxymorphone	Opana Numorphan,	Biscuits, Blue Heaven, Blues, Mrs. O, O Bomb, Octagons, Stop Signs	Tablets	Swallowed, snorted, injected	
Tapentadol	Nucynta, Tapal, Palexia	Cha Cha	Oral suspension, tablets	Swallowed, snorted, injected	II
Tramadol	Ultram©, Ultracet, ConZip, Ryzolt, Rybix ODT and	Chill Pills, Ultras	Tablets, capsules	Swallowed, snorted injected	III

OVER THE COUNTER DRUGS					
GENERIC NAMES	**TRADE NAMES**	**STREET NAMES**	**APPEARANCES**	**ROUTE OF INGESTION**	**SCHEDULE**
Dextromethorphan	Many: Vicks 44, Creomulsion, Delsym, Tussin Pediatric, DM	Robotripping, Robo, Skittles, Triple C, DXM, Syrup,	Syrup, Tablets	Oral, syrup injection	N
Kratom	No commercial name	Herbal Speedball, Biak-biak, Ketum, Kahuam, Ithang, Thom.	Fresh or dried leaves, powder, liquid, gum	Chewed (whole leaves), eaten (mixed in food or brewed as tea), occasionally smoked	N
Loperamide	Imodium	None	Tablet, capsule, liquid	Swallowed	N
Inhalants	Various	Poppers, Snappers, Whippets, Laughing gas	Paint thinners or removers, degreasers, dry cleaning fluids, gasoline, lighter fluids, correction fluids, permanent markers, electronic cleaners and freeze sprays, glue, spray paint, hair or deodorant sprays, fabric protector sprays, aerosol computer cleaning products, vegetable oil sprays, butane lighter, propane tanks, whipped cream aerosol containers, refrigerant gases, ether, chloroform, halothane, nitrous oxide	Inhaled through the nose and mouth	N

HALLUCINOGENS					
GENERIC NAMES	**TRADE NAMES**	**STREET NAMES**	**APPEARANCES**	**ROUTE OF INGESTION**	**SCHEDULE**
Alcohol	Wine, Beer, Liquor	Booze, Brew	Color or colorless liquid	Oral	N
Dextromethorphan	Many: Vicks 44, Creomulsion, Delsym, Tussin Pediatric, DM	Robotripping, Robo, Skittles, Triple C, DXM, Syrup,	Syrup, Tablets	Oral, syrup injection	N
Ketamine	Ketalar	Super K, Kit-Kat, Kitty, Special K, Vitamin K, Cat Valium	White powder, clear or cream-colored liquid	Injected, mixed in beverage, sniffed, snorted, smoked (powder added to tobacco or marijuana cigarettes), swallowed	III
Lysergic Acid Diethylamide (LSD)	Delysid	Acid, Dots, Window Panes, Blotter, Blue Heaven, Cubes, Microdot, Yellow Sunshine, Sugar Cubes	White, odorless powder, tablets, capsules, solids, liquids, sugar cubes, gelatin, blotting paper	Oral	I
Mescaline (Peyote)	None	Mesc, Cactus, Buttons	Natural-looking fresh or dried "buttons", tablets or capsules	Oral, Chewed, nasal, smoked, injected	I
Phencyclidine (PCP)	Sernyl, Sernylan	Angel Dust, boat Space Cadet, Pcp, Hog Dust, White Devil, peace pill	White or colored powder, tablets or capsules, colorless crystals, clear liquid	Oral, nasal, smoked, swallowed, injected. Added to marijuana, mint	I

CANNABINOIDS					
GENERIC NAMES	TRADE NAMES	STREET NAMES	APPEARANCES	ROUTE OF INGESTION	SCHEDULE
Cannabis, Marijuana, Hashish	Marinol, Dronabinol	Blunt, Bud, Dope, Ganja, Grass, Green, Herb, Joint, Mary Jane, Pot, Reefer, Sinsemilla, Skunk, Smoke, Trees, Weed; Hashish: Boom, Gangster, Hash, Hemp	Seeds, oils, leaves, capsules, buds, liquid	Mixed in food or teat, smoked, oral	I
Synthetic Cannabinoids	JWH-018, UR-144, XLR-11 (5-F-UR144), AB-PINACA, 5-F-AB-PINACA, AB-CHMINACA, APP-CHMINACA, AB-FUBINACA, AB-CHMICA, ADBICA, and 5-F-ABICA to name a few	K2, Spice Gold, Spice, Sdiamond, Yucatan Fire, Genie, Fire N Ice, Black Mamba, Bombay Blue, Zombie World, The Moon, Bliss	Powder, plant extracts	Snorted, smoked, sold as incense, potpourri	I

MUSCLE RELAXANT					
GENERIC NAMES	TRADE NAMES	STREET NAMES	APPEARANCES	ROUTE OF INGESTION	SCHEDULE
Carisoprodol	Soma, Prosoma	Ds, Dance, Las Vegas Cocktail	Pills	Bumped, injected, smoked	IV

CENTRAL NERVOUS SYSTEM STIMULANTS					
GENERIC NAMES	**TRADE NAMES**	**STREET NAMES**	**APPEARANCES**	**ROUTE OF INGESTION**	**SCHEDULE**
Amphetamine	Adderall, Benzedrine, Dexedrine	Bennies, Black Beauties, Crosses, Hearts, LA Turnaround, Speed, Truck Drivers, Uppers	Tablets, capsules, solution	Oral, nasal, smoked, injected	II
Bath Salts	Cathinone, Methylenedioxypyro valerone, Mephedrone	Flakka, Ivory Wave, Plant Fertilizer, Vanilla Sky, Energy-1, Red Dove, White Dove, Blue Silk, Zoom, Hurricane, Aura, Alpha PVC	White, tan, or brown colored powdery substance	Ingested, snorted, smoked, or injected	I
Cocaine	None	Blow, Rock Bump, Coke, Snow, Crack, Flake, Toot, Cola, White Girl	White Powder, whitish rock crystal	Oral, nasal smoked, injected	II
Ecstasy/MDMA	None	Peace, Uppers, Lovers Speed, Ecstasy, X-Tc, Adam, Skittles, Tabs, Molly	Colorful tabs, liquid, white powder, capsules, tablets	Oral, injected, snorted.	I
Methamphetamine	Desoxyn, Methedrine	Crank, Glass Doe, Crystal, Speed, Ice, Meth, Tina	Tablets, capsules, solution, crystal meth glass, white powder	Oral, smoked, nasal, injected	II
Methylphenidate	Ritalin, Concerta	JIF, MPH, Skippy, The Smart Drug, Vitamin R, Diet Coke, Kiddy Coke, R Pop, Study, Pineapple, Poor Man's Cocaine,	Tablets, capsules, patches, and liquid	Snorted, smoked, Oral (dissolve in beverage) Chewed, injected	II

CENTRAL NERVOUS SYSTEM DEPRESSANTS					
GENERIC NAMES	TRADE NAMES	STREET NAMES	APPEARANCES	ROUTE OF INGESTION	SCHEDULE
BARBITURATES:					
Amobarbital	Amytal, Stadadorm	Barbs, Blues, Blue Dolls, Rainbows, Nebbies, Downers, Reds, Red Devils, Phennies, Red Birds, Reds, Tooies, Yellow Jackets, Yellows	Capsule, powder, tablets, solution	Swallowed snorted, injected	II, III, IV
Butabarbital	Butisol				
Butalbital	Fiorinal				
Pentobarbital	Luminal, Neodorm				
Phenobarbital	Nembutal				
Secobarbital	Seconal				
BENZODIAZEPINE:					
Alprazolam	Xanax	Candy, Benzo, Bzd, Nerve Pills, Goofballs, Valley Girl, Heavenly Blues, Stupefy , Downers, Sleeping Pills, Tranks	Capsule, powder, tablets, solution	Swallowed snorted, injected	IV
Chlordiazepoxide	Librium				
Clonazepam	Klonopin				
Clorazepate	Tranxene				
Diazepam	Valium				
Flurazepam	Dalmane				
Lorazepam	Ativan, Tavor, Tamestra				
Oxazepam	Serax				
Temazepam	Restoril				
Triazolam	Halcion				
ROHYPNOL (Flunitrazepam)	Flunitrazepam, Rohypnol®	Circles, Date Rape Drug, Forget Pill, Forget-Me Pill, La Rocha, Lunch Money, Mexican Valium, Mind Eraser, Pingus, R2, Reynolds, Rib, Roach, Roach 2, Roaches, Roachies, Roapies, Rochas Dos, Roofies, Rope, Rophies, Row-shay, Ruffies, Trip-and-Fall, Wolfies	Tablet	Swallowed (as a pill or as dissolved in a drink), snorted, injected	IV

Reference

National Institute on Drug Abuse. Commonly abused drugs charts-

https://www.drugabuse.gov/drugs-abuse/commonly-abused-drugs-charts Accessed April 2, 2018.

CHAPTER FOUR

Useful Resources and Websites

 U.S. Department of Health & Human Services (HHS) function to enhance and protect the health and well-being of all Americans. It is the government's principal agency for protecting the health and well-being of all Americans.
 https://www.hhs.gov/HHS.gov: About the Opioid Epidemic
https://www.hhs.gov/opioids/about-the-epidemic/

Centers for Medicare and Medicaid (CMS) is responsible for overseeing most of the regulations that are related directly to the healthcare system. It is a federal agency within the United States Department of Health and Human Services.
https://www.cms.gov/

Centers for Disease Control and Prevention (CDC): working 24/7 seven to protect Americans from health and safety threats both foreign and domestic.
800-CDC-INFO (800-232-4636) TTY: 888-232-6348
Email CDC-INFO   https://www.cdc.gov

SAMHSA - Substance Abuse and Mental Health Services Administration SAMHSA's mission is to reduce the impact of substance abuse and mental illness on America's communities. Congress established the Substance Abuse and Mental Health Services Administration (**SAMHSA**) in 1992 to make substance use and mental disorder information, services, and research more accessible. **https://www.samhsa.gov/**
SAMHSA's Behavioral Health Treatment Services Locator
SAMHSA website (*www.dpt.samhsa.gov*)

National Institute of Health (NIH), a part of the U.S. Department of Health and Human Services, is the nation's medical research agency — making important discoveries that improve health and save lives.
https://www.nih.gov/about-nih/who-we-are

National Institute on Drug Abuse (NIDA), an institute of NIH. The mission of the National Institute on Drug Abuse (NIDA) is to advance science on the causes and consequences of drug use and addiction and to apply that knowledge to improve individual and public health.
https://www.drugabuse.gov/

The Food and Drug Administration (FDA), Mission; The Food and Drug Administration is responsible for protecting the public health by ensuring the safety, efficacy, and security of human and veterinary drugs, biological products, and medical devices; and by ensuring the safety of our nation's food supply, cosmetics, and products that emit radiation. Mar 28, 2018.
https://www.fda.gov/aboutfda/whatwedo/default.htm

The Drug Enforcement Administration (DEA): controlled substance laws and regulations and aims to reduce the supply of and demand for such substances.
https://www.usa.gov/federal-agencies/drug-enforcement-administration

The Agency for Healthcare Research and Quality (AHRQ), its mission is to produce evidence to make health care safer, higher quality, more accessible, equitable, and affordable, and to work within the U.S. Department of Health and Human Services and with other partners to make sure that the evidence is understood and used. https://www.ahrq.gov/cpi/about/mission/index.html

The Joint Commission–The Joint Commission accredits and certifies
healthcare organizations and programs in the United States that have met the standard of care as set by the commission.
https://www.jointcommission.org/certification/certification_main.aspx

The National Committee for Quality Assurance (NCQA) – "exists to improve the quality of health care. **We work for better healthcare, better choices and better health"**
https://www.ncqa.org/

The Office of National Drug Control Policy (ONDCP).

Works to reduce drug use and its consequences by leading and coordinating the development, implementation, and assessment of US drug policy

in addition to its vital ongoing work, ONDCP also provides

administrative and financial support to the President's Commission

on Combating Drug Addiction and the Opioid Crisis.

https://www.whitehouse.gov/ondcp/

The Environmental Protection Agency (EPA)

Mission is to protect human health and the environment.

https://www.epa.gov/aboutepa/our-mission-and-what-we-do

Psychiatry

American Academy of Addiction Psychiatry website (*www.aaap.org*)

The National Alliance on Mental Illness, (NAMI), **https://www.nami.org**
3803 N. Fairfax Drive, Suite 100 Arlington, VA 22203. Main 703-524-7600
Member Services 888-999-6264, Help Line 800-950-6264

To report SUSPECTED ADVERSE EVENTS, contact:
The manufacturer of the product taken or FDA MedWatch program by phone at 1-800-FDA-1088 or online at www.fda.gov/medwatch/repor
Treatment

For information on buprenorphine treatment, contact the SAMHSA Center for Substance Abuse Treatment (CSAT) at 866-BUP-CSAT (866-287-2728) or infobuprenorphine@samhsa.hhs.gov (link sends e-mail).

For information about other medication-assisted treatment (MAT) or the certification of opioid treatment programs (OTPs), contact the SAMHSA Division of Pharmacologic Therapies at 240-276-2700 or otp-extranet@opioid.samhsa.gov (link sends e-mail).

Contact SAMHSA's regional OTP Compliance Officers to determine if an OTP is qualified to provide treatment for substance use disorder

https://www.cdc.gov/vitalsigns/heroin/index.html

American Society of Addiction Medicine, website: *www.asam.org*

For more information about drug addiction treatment,
 visit:www.drugabuse.gov/publications/principles-drug-addiction-treatment-research-based-guide-third-edition/acknowledgments

For information about **drug addiction treatment in the criminal justice system**, visit: www.drugabuse.gov/publications/principles-drug-abuse-treatment-criminal-justice-populations/principles

For step-by-step guides for people who think they or a loved one may need treatment, visit: www.drugabuse.gov/related-topics/treatment

Naloxone

For general information about your state's policies regarding naloxone, see the following online resources: • Naloxone Overdose Prevention Laws Database; Database from the Prescription Drug http://pdaps.org/datasets/laws-regulating-administration-of-naloxone-1501695139

Abuse Policy System website. http://pdaps.org/

This database, in the form of an interactive US map from the Prescription Drug Abuse Policy System website, allows users to look up naloxone access laws by state. As of October 2017, the site covers laws passed from 1/1/01 to 7/1/17.

• Legal Interventions to Reduce Overdose Mortality: Naloxone Access and Overdose
Good Samaritan Laws.

This fact sheet, from the Network for Public Health Law website, provides a comprehensive table of naloxone access policies by state as of July 15, 2017.

http://www.ncsl.org/research/civil-and-criminal-justice/drug-overdose-immunity-good-samaritan-laws.aspx

Some Medical and Professional Associations

- Academy of PM& R (AAPM&R)
  http://www.aapmr.org/education/me
- American College of Sports Medicine
- National Stroke Association
- Neurosurgeon.com
- American Association of Neuromuscular and Electrodiagnostic Medicine
- Academic Orthopedic Society
- American Academy of Orthopedic Surgeons
- American Academy of Family Medicine
- Spine Intervention Society https://www.spineintervention.org
- American Academy of Pain Medicine
- National American Spine Society
- American Academy of Pediatrics
- American Academy of Neurological Surgeons
- American Medical Association
- American Society for Surgery
- American Society of Internal Medicine
- Society of General Internal Medicine
- Radiological Society of North America
- American Academy of Neurology
- American Board of Pain Medicine. http://www.abpm.org
- American Society of Interventional Pain Physicians:
  http://www.asipp.org/default.html
- American Chiropractic Association https://www.acatoday.org/
- American Dental Association   https://www.ada.org/
- American Physical Therapy Association http://www.apta.org/
- American Society of Addiction Medicine https://www.asam.org/

Other Useful Sites

> - **Alcoholic Anonymous   https://www.aa.org/**
> - **Harm Reduction Coalition** - https://harmreduction.org/
> - **The National Domestic Hotline** https://www.thehotline.org/
> - **National Suicide Prevention Lifeline** https://suicidepreventionlifeline.org/
> - **Help and Resources | Drug Overdose | CDC Injury Center** https://www.cdc.gov/drugoverdose/prevention/help.html
> - **Narcotic Anonymous** https://www.na.org/

CONCLUSION

The opioid epidemic will be around for a while and during that time will create significant damage and have an immense impact on our society as we know it now. However, even when there is no epidemic and opioids are no longer one of the main focus of our society, the need for opioids as effective medications for pain control among other things will still be here.

The opioid epidemic is real, and just like all the other drugs or substance abuse issues, unfortunately, it is not going anywhere fast. It will evolve, it can and will change for the better we all hope. However, one of the sad truths is that it has a significant potential to get even worse.

FOCAS is a classification that has the potential to stand the test of time, regardless of the extent of use of opioids. Its use will allow common nomenclatures in healthcare with regards to opioids use and addiction treatment. It is not a perfect classification, as indicated they are overlaps in its application, but there are many similarities when compared with other classifications that were implemented or used.

INDEX

ABOUT THE AUTHOR

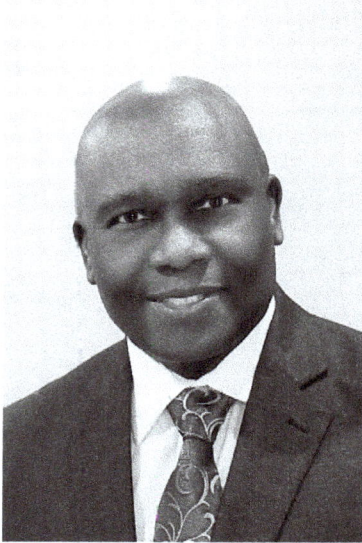

D Terrence Foster, M.D., MA, FAAPMR, DABPM

Dr. Foster graduated from The Albert Einstein College of Medicine of Yeshiva University, New York, where he earned his Doctor of Medicine. At the City University of New York, he received a Master's Degree in Chemistry and from the University of the West Indies, a Bachelor of Science - BS (Hons) in Chemistry. His medical training was completed at Jacobi Medical Center/Albert Einstein Hospital, New York - Internship. Residency at New York University Medical Center/ Rusk Institute of Rehabilitation Medicine-Physical Medicine & Rehabilitation and Medical College of Wisconsin, Milwaukee: Fellowship, Electrodiagnostic Medicine (EMG).

Dr. Foster worked as an Attending Physician and Clinical Instructor at Emory University Hospitals, Wesley Woods Geriatric Hospital and Center for Rehab Medicine. He is a former Medical Director for The Rehabilitation Center at Southern Regional Health System, Riverdale, GA, where he served for ten years.

Dr. Foster has medical staff privileges at several medical centers in the state of Georgia. He is currently the Medical Director for the Center for Pain and Rehab Medicine in Stockbridge, GA, where his primary focus is Interventional Pain and Addiction Medicine.

He is Board Certified in Physical Medicine and Rehabilitation, and a fellow of the American Academy of Physical Medicine and Rehabilitation. He is also a Diplomate of the American Board of Physical Medicine and Rehabilitation. He is Board Certified in Pain Medicine and a Diplomate of the American Board of Pain Medicine.

Dr. Foster is the author or co-author of several scientific articles and the author of the book *The Opioid Epidemic Consumers & HealthCare Guide.* He also previously hosted a radio show called "The Doctor Show." He is a member of several medical associations.

Visit his website at DTERRENCEFOSTER.COM
Photo by: Atlanta Photographers Network.

ANOTHER   BOOK   BY DR. D TERRENCE FOSTER

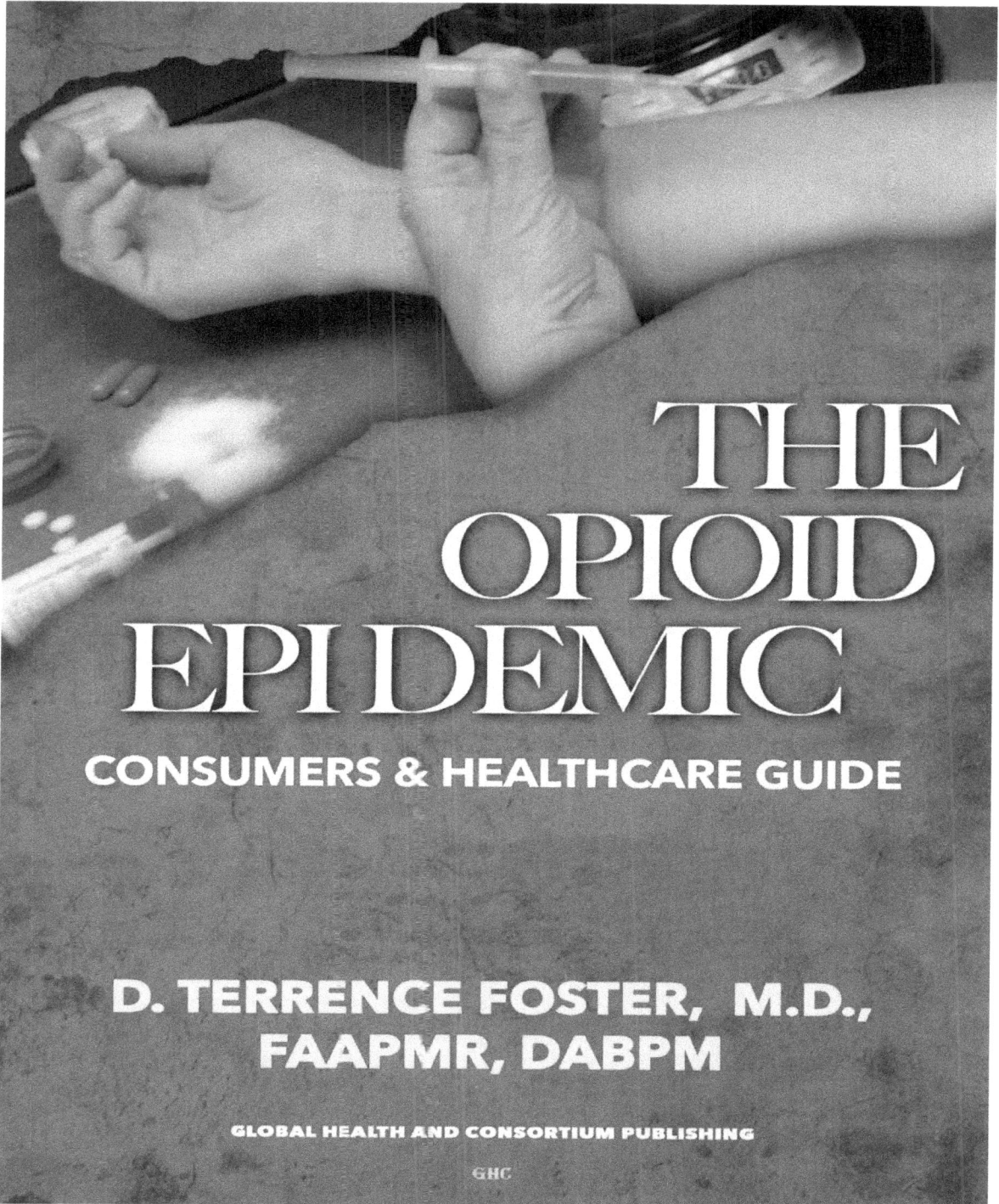

THE OPIOID EPIDEMIC

CONSUMERS & HEALTHCARE GUIDE

D. TERRENCE FOSTER, M.D., FAAPMR, DABPM

GLOBAL HEALTH AND CONSORTIUM PUBLISHING

GHC

NOTES

D. TERRENCE FOSTER, M.D.

NOTES

NOTES

D. TERRENCE FOSTER, M.D.

NOTES

NOTES

www.ingramcontent.com/pod-product-compliance
Lightning Source LLC
Chambersburg PA
CBHW081658270326
41933CB00017B/3208